LITTLE BOOK OF

PILATES

LITTLE BOOK OF
PILATES

First published in the UK in 2013

© Demand Media Limited 2014

www.demand-media.co.uk

Printed and bound in Europe.

ISBN 978-1-782811-81-7

Contents

Introduction

Pilates is a physical fitness system developed in the early 20th century by Joseph Pilates whose concept was intended to strengthen the human mind and body. Pilates believed that mental and physical health is interrelated. It is an extremely popular method of exercise all over the world. Pilates called his method 'Contrology' from the word 'control'.

The techniques employed for Pilates builds up flexibility, muscle strength, and endurance in the legs, abdominals, arms, hips and back. It puts emphasis on spinal and pelvic alignment, breathing and developing a strong core, as well as improving coordination and balance. The Pilates' method allows for different exercises to be modified in range of difficulty from beginner to advanced. Intensity of exercises can therefore be increased over time as the body conditions and adapts to the exercises.

The Little Book of Pilates features hand-picked exercises chosen to help you achieve the bottom that you have only dreamed about before. The Body Control Pilates Method is highly effective for everyone, regardless of whether you are new to Pilates or already a regular participant. These specially selected exercises will be the perfect addition to your normal exercise routines.

This book features Lynne Robinson, the world's most popular Pilates teacher. Her programme Pilates the Bottom Line is also available on DVD to complement this volume.

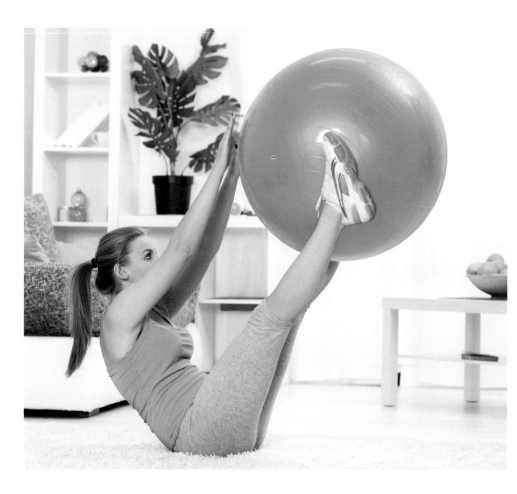

LITTLE BOOK OF **PILATES**

DO NOT EXERCISE:

If you are feeling at all unwell, as it is counter-productive.

If you have eaten a heavy meal in the past two hours.

If you have been drinking alcohol.

If you are in pain from an injury, consult your doctor first, as rest may be needed before you exercise.

If you have taken painkillers as they will mask any warning pains.

If you are undergoing medical treatment or taking any drugs, you will need to consult your doctor first.

Remember it is always wise to consult your doctor before you take up a new exercise regime, and always stop an exercise it if causes pain.

Although many of these exercises are fine for use in pregnancy, we cannot recommend that you follow them as the book has not been written with pregnancy in mind.

Chapter 1

Spine Curls into Bridge

Start with an ordinary spine curl. For this, lie on the mat with your knees bent and have your feet together, otherwise you are still in the relaxation position. Have your arms by your sides, your elbows softly open and just lengthen through the fingertips.

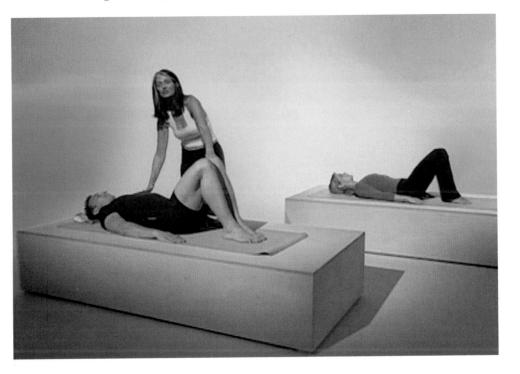

SPINE CURLS INTO BRIDGE

Take a deep breath in to prepare and as you breathe out you zip up the pelvic floor, squeeze your buttocks and slowly, bone by bone, peel the spine up from the mat.

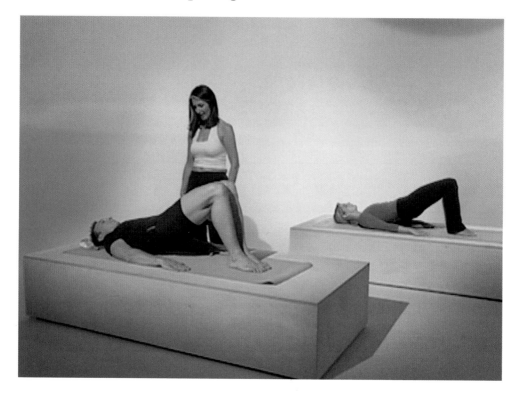

Breathe in deeply at the top and as you breathe out, one by one, replace the vertebrae back down, zipping the whole time and coming back to the neutral position.

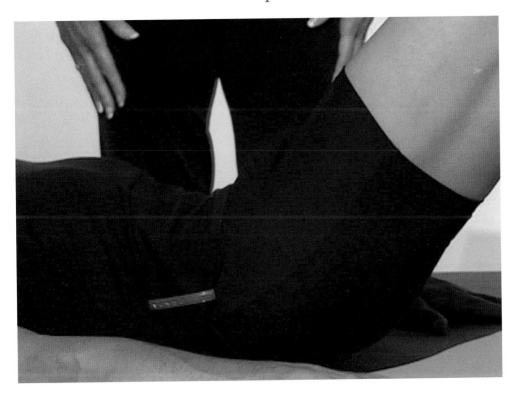

Moving into the bridge position: take a deep breath in to prepare again, zip up the pelvis and squeeze the buttocks. Curl the tailbone up and slowly, bone by bone, peel the spine up from the mat. Stay in this position and you need to work your buttocks a little bit harder: breathe in and as you breathe out straighten one leg, keeping it in line with the other knee. Breathe in and bend it back down, breathe out and straighten the other leg and then bring it back down.

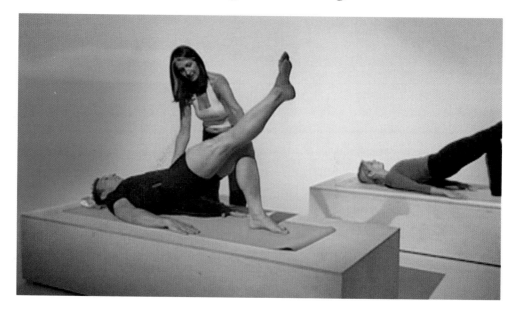

Breathe in and as you breathe out, one by one, replace the vertebrae back down, zipping the whole time and coming back to the neutral position.

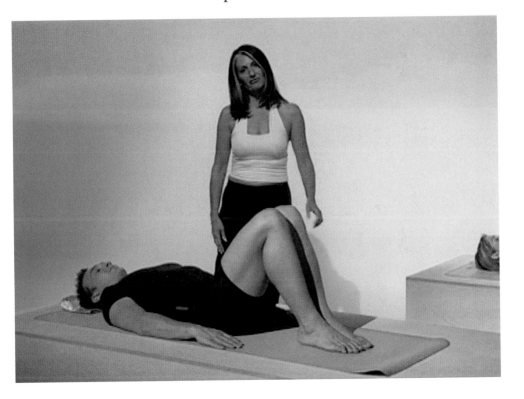

A more advanced version can also be performed: as before, take a deep breath in to prepare and as you breathe out zip up the pelvic floor, squeeze your buttocks and slowly, bone by bone, peel the spine up from the mat. Breathe in and float the arms up bringing them in line with your ears. As you breathe out straighten one leg keeping the pelvis absolutely level.

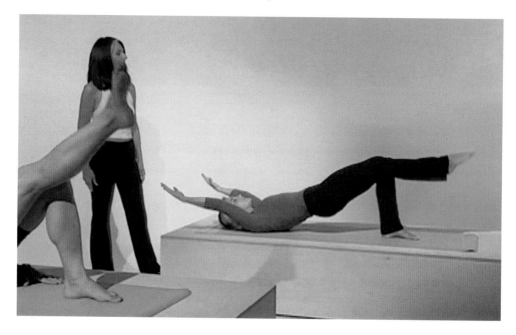

Breathe in and fold the leg down again. Breathe out and straighten the other leg. Then slowly spine curl back down. Finish by bringing your arms back down by your sides. Repeat twice more.

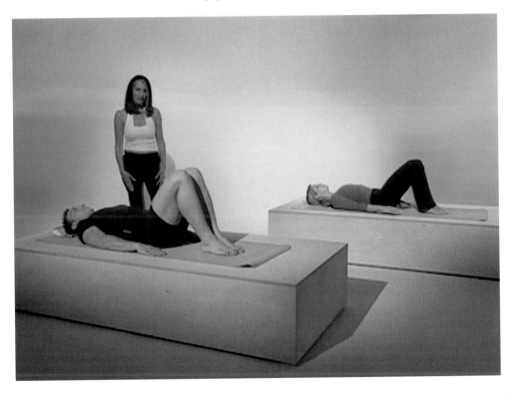

Chapter 2

Bridging

Bridging works on your pelvic and lumbar stability and you may find that you're more comfortable without a pillow for this exercise. You may also find that you're more comfortable with your feet hip width apart; some people find it easier in this position, others with their feet together. Experiment until you get the most comfortable version for you.

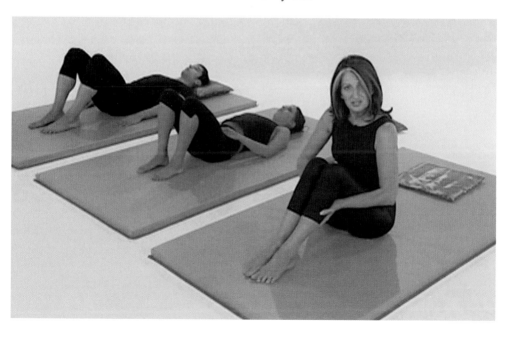

Lie on the mat, with or without your head cushion. Take a moment to allow the spine to lengthen and to find the neutral position. Hold your pelvis lightly to ensure that your pelvis stays level when you come up into the bridge position. Breathe in deeply and straighten one leg first making sure that your pelvis stays level.

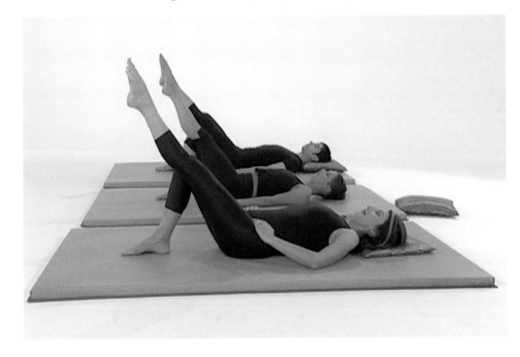

On the out breath, zip up the pelvis and slowly curl up. Breathe in, breathe out and bend the knee back down and slowly curl back down. Repeat with the other leg.

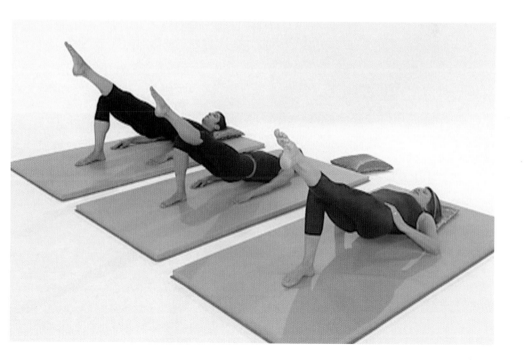

To make this a bit harder repeat the exercise but this time, once you have curled your spine up, take your raised leg higher and point your toes towards the ceiling. Do not let your pelvis dip. Breathe in and on the out breath lower the leg then bend the knee back down and slowly curl back down. Repeat with the other leg.

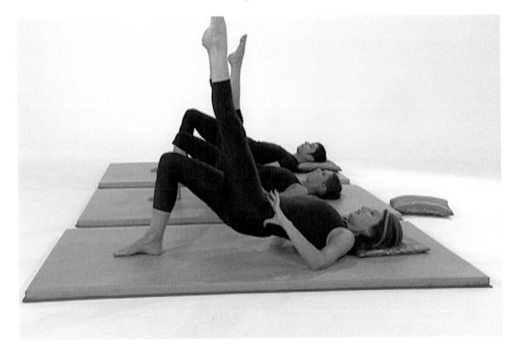

The last version of this exercise is to curl up into the bridge position without straightening the leg first. Then breathe in and as you breathe out extend the leg, and on the next out breath, raise the leg to the ceiling.

Step 1

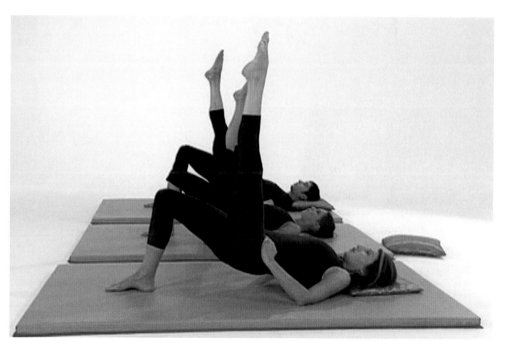

Then take the leg down to the floor but without allowing the pelvis to dip.

Step 2

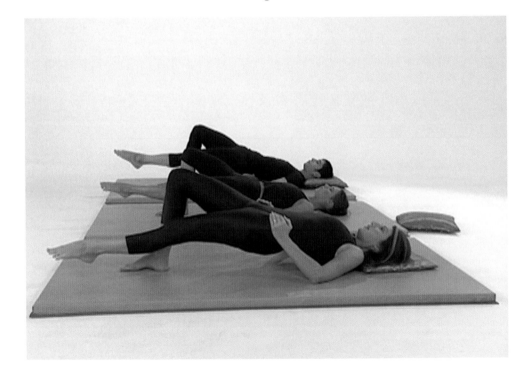

Bring the leg back up to level, then bend the knee back down and slowly curl back down. Repeat on the other leg.

Step 3

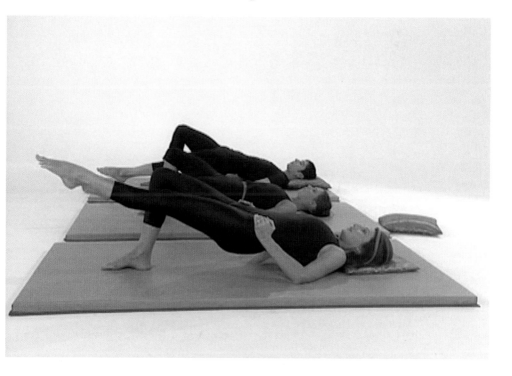

Chapter 3

The Oyster

The Oyster really targets a deep buttock muscle and for this you need to be lying on your side with your head resting on your extended arm, shoulder over shoulder, hip over hip, knee over knee and your feet stacked one on top of the other in a line with your bottom – don't take them too far behind or in front of you.

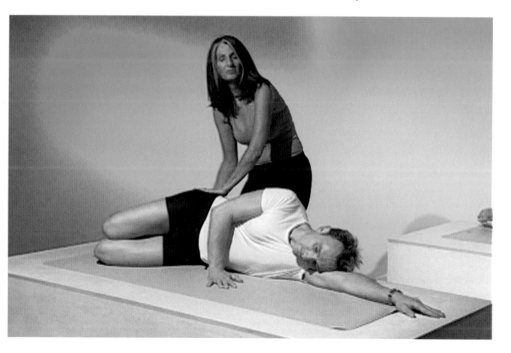

Throughout the whole exercise you need to be lifting from your waist, keeping it nice and long and lengthening through the spine.

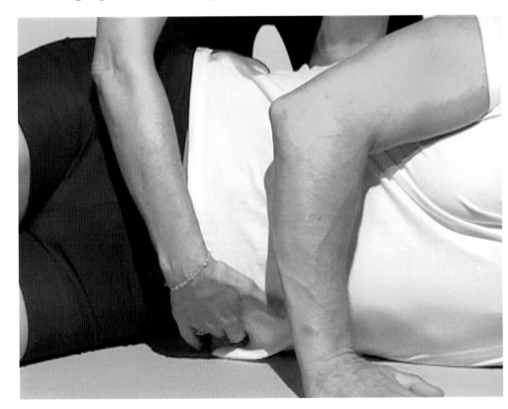

Oyster 1: take a deep breath in and as you breathe out zip up the pelvis and slowly, keeping your feet together, open the top knee making sure that the top hip doesn't roll back. Breathe in and lower. Repeat five times on that side (you can work up to doing ten).

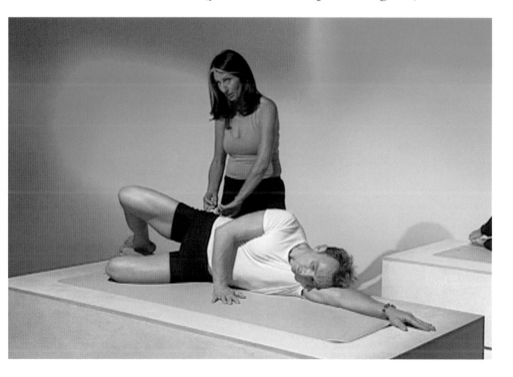

A variation on this is Oyster 2: for this, the feet are going to lift off as well. Breathe in and as you breathe out zip up the pelvis and open the top knee and lift the feet at the same time. Breathe in and lower. Repeat this three times.

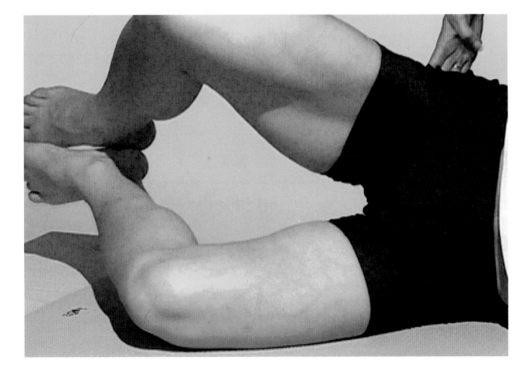

A more advanced version of this is called Boxes: from the Oyster position, bring your knees forward, just soft of 90 degrees in a chair-like position.

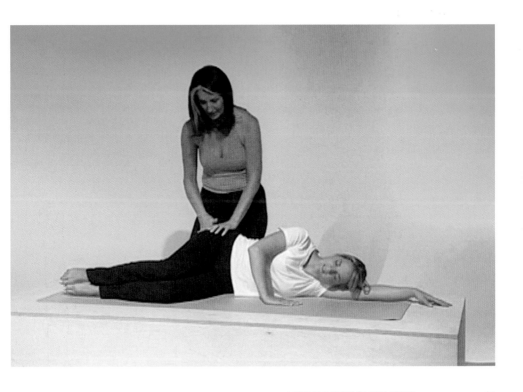

Breathe in and as you breathe out zip up the pelvis, lengthen the top leg so that it is in line with your body and with toes pointed.

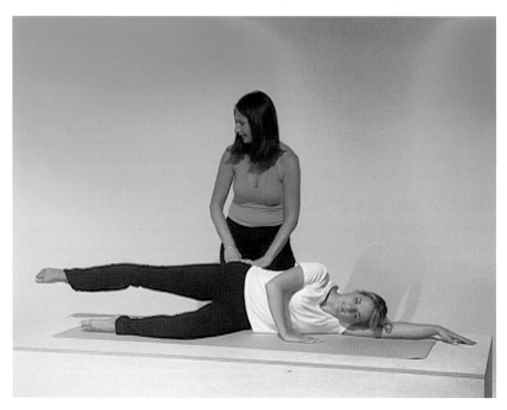

You need to draw a box with your leg, so breathe in and as you breathe out bring the leg in front of you a little. Lift it a little – about six inches – and as you breathe out, take it back behind you (but without letting your back arch) then lower it, then bring it in front again, lift again then take it back. The movements are all quite small and you are drawing a box with your foot. Repeat five times.

Step 1

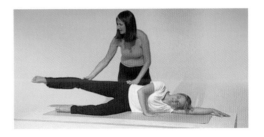

Step 2

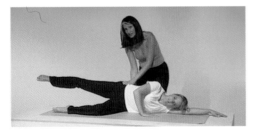

Step 3

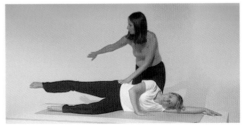

Turn onto your other side and repeat Oyster 1, Oyster 2 and Boxes.

Chapter 4

Abductor Lifts

For this exercise you can wear leg weights, which can weigh up to about two and a half pounds each weight. It is recommended that you start without using any weights at all and build up to using this weight. If you haven't got any leg weights, you can easily make your own by taking a pair of tights, cut off the legs and pour in some rice or something similar depending on what weight you want. Tie the ends and then the weight is ready to be wrapped around your leg.

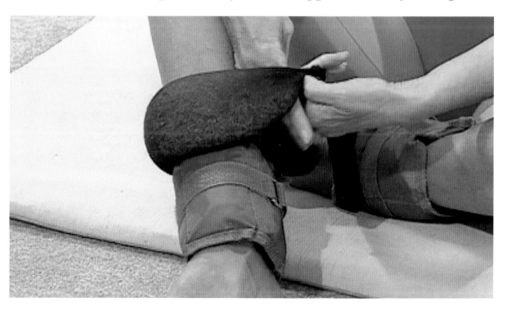

Your position for this exercise is really important and you'll want an extra cushion to hand for later on. Lie on the mat and line yourself up with the edge of your mat so that your back is nice and straight. Have one knee over the other and at a right angle with your body and with your feet, knees and hips lined up. Pelvis square and with a pillow under your head so that your neck is comfortable. Your arm should be in a straight line with your body.

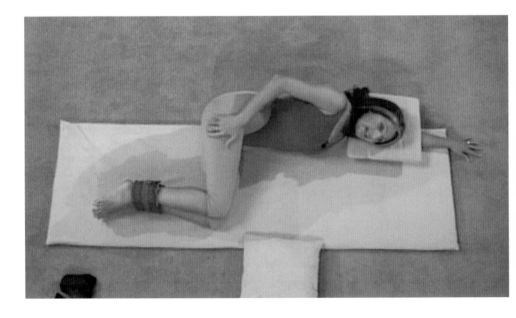

As you breathe out raise your leg about six inches and lower it to hip height as you breathe in. Repeat ten times.

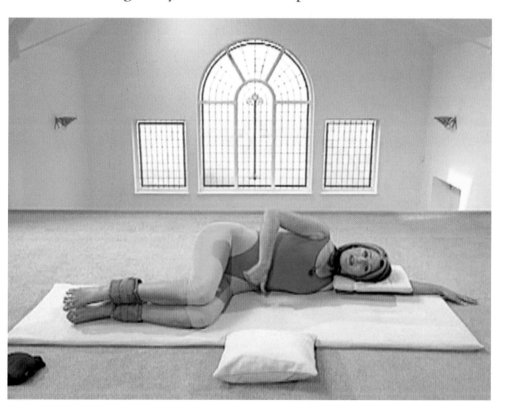

To work the buttocks and outer thigh: breathe in and breathe out, zip up your pelvis then straighten the top leg so that it's in line with your hip and body. Lengthen through from the tips of your fingers right through to your heel. Flex the foot.

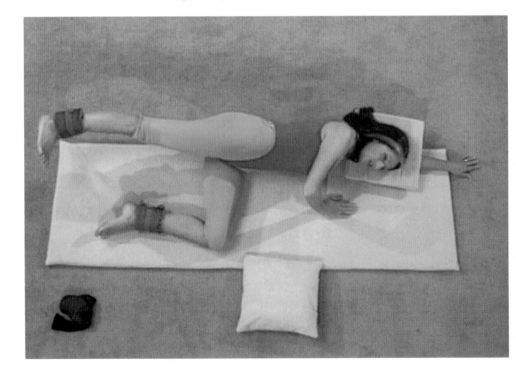

Step 1

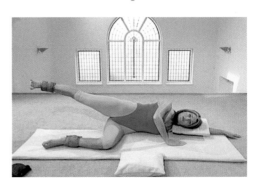

Throughout the exercise you need to be lifting your waist up off the floor and zipping up the pelvis, as well as thinking about having a very long waist. Place your other hand in front of you to steady you with your top shoulder blade down and back in line with your other shoulder – as if you're lying with a brick wall behind you.

Step 2

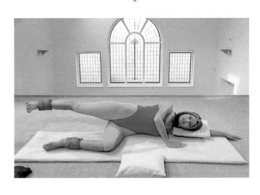

Bend the knee and place it back on top of the other leg.

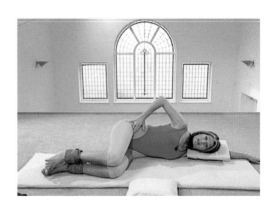

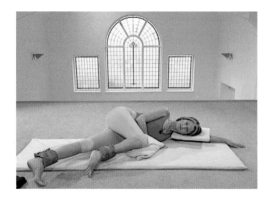

To work the inside of the thigh: place your second cushion underneath your top knee in a cocked position. As you do so make sure that you don't allow your pelvis to roll forward; it has to be completely square with one hipbone over the other. Stretch the bottom leg away from you with the foot flexed and turn the leg out from the hip.

Breathe in and breathe out and zip up the pelvis. Slowly raise the bottom leg and lower as you breathe in. Repeat ten times.

Step 1

Step 2

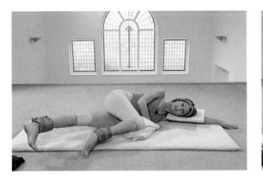
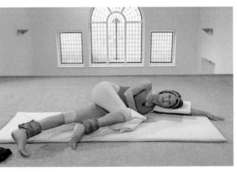

Repeat all of the above on the other side.

Chapter 5

Front and Back

Lie on your side, stacking up all your joints one on top of the other. Rest your head on your elbow if you can, or, if this is uncomfortable take your head down so that it rests on your arm instead.

Step 1

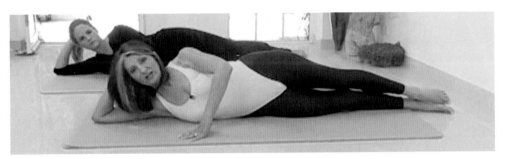

Step 2

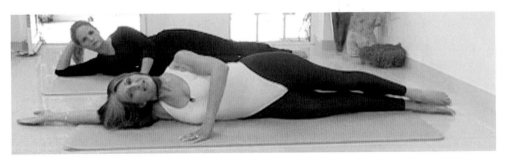

Bring both legs forward by about 45 degrees to give you a bit more stability with your top hand in front of you for extra support.

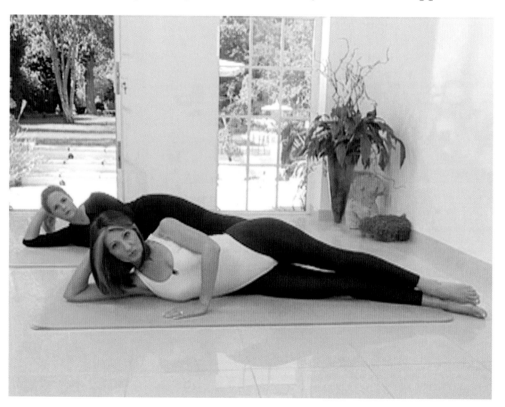

Take a breath in and as you breathe out bring your top leg up to hip height and then in front of you, hinging from the hip.

Step 1

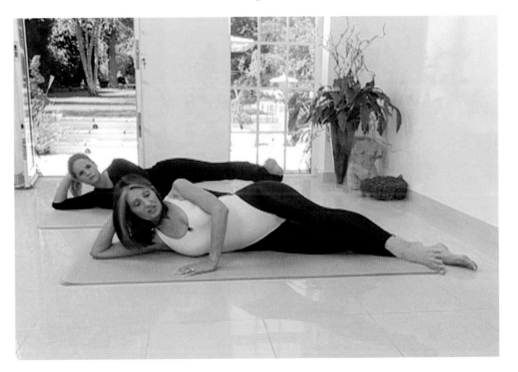

Then take the leg behind you on the out breath making sure that the pelvis doesn't roll or move back – keep it very still.

Step 2

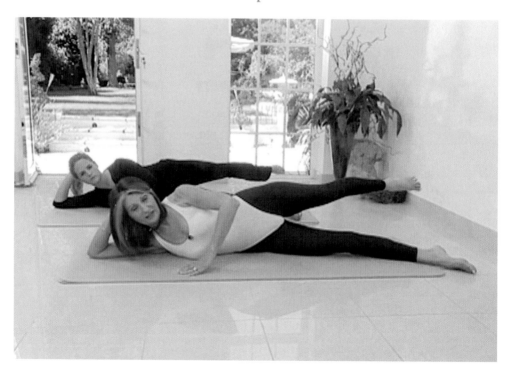

Once you are used to the movement try flexing the foot on the forward
movement. Repeat this six times and then repeat on the other side.

Step 3

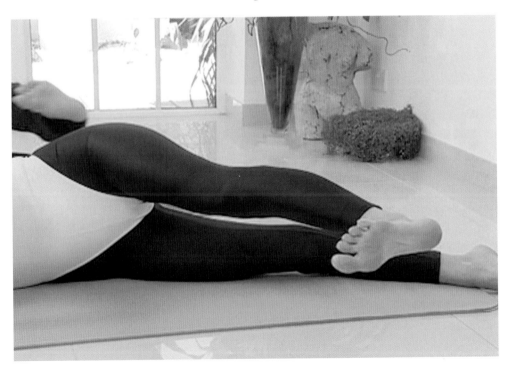

Chapter 6

Star Circles

Lying on your front, take your hands and fold them underneath your forehead. Have your legs just wider than hip width apart and make five very small circles with your leg by raising it off the ground a little and then repeat in the opposite direction. Make sure that both hips stay on the mat and the pelvis is zipped and stays square. Repeat on the other side.

Step 1

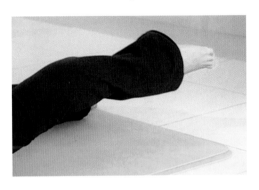

Step 2

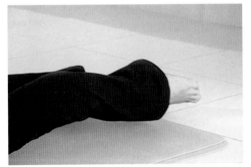

Step 3

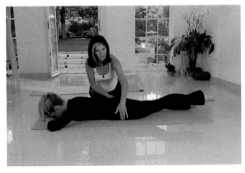

Chapter 7

Grasshopper

Lying on your front, take your hands and fold them underneath your forehead. Have your legs just wider than hip width apart and lift both legs this time. Then beat your heels together for a count of five as you breathe in and a count of five as you breathe out. Repeat twice more.

Step 1

Step 2

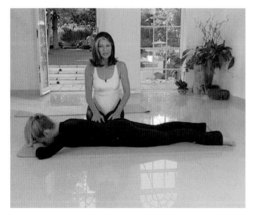

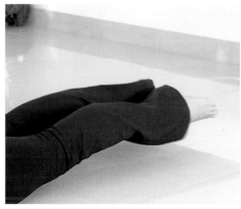

Chapter 8

Back Stretch

Kneel on all fours with your hands beneath your shoulders and knees beneath your hips, and with your pelvis and spine in the neutral position, neck nice and long. Bring your feet together but leave your knees apart, and slowly lower yourself back down. Rest your forehead onto the mat and stretch out taking a few deep breaths. Hold the stretch for about twenty seconds. Avoid this exercise if you have a knee injury.

Step 1

Step 2

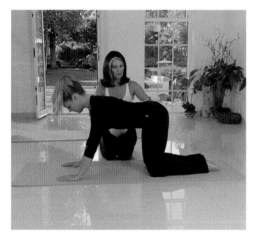
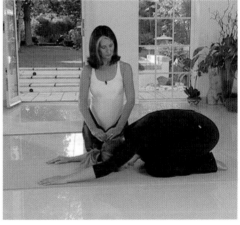

As you breathe out for the last time, bone by bone, bring your pubic bone forward as you slowly roll back up through the spine.

Step 1

Step 2

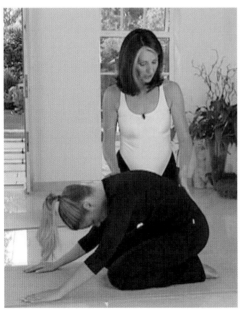
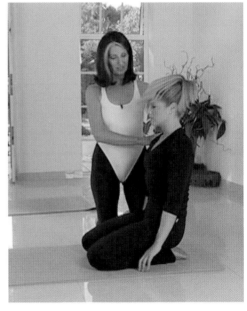

Chapter 9

Single Leg Kicks

Lie on your front with your hands under your forehead and legs together. Squeezing your inner thighs together throughout, kick one leg in and as that leg goes down, kick the other leg in. The legs do not go down onto the mat but stay just off it. Repeat five times on each leg. Add a small pulse of two counts as each leg comes in and repeat again for five.

Step 1

Step 2

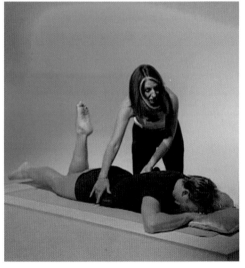

A more advanced version of the above is to do the same as above but come up onto your elbows with your hands made into fists with your pubic bone pushed into the mat. Push slightly into the forearms as you do the legs and this will work the upper arms as well.

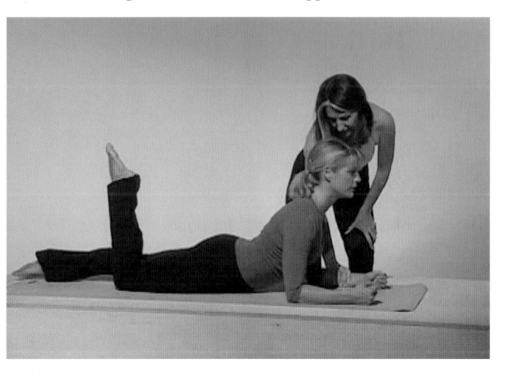

Chapter 10

Table Top

One of the hardest things to get right about this exercise is your alignment, so if you can do it next to a mirror all the better.

Come onto all fours with your hands directly beneath your shoulders and your knees beneath your hips. Look straight down and keep your neck nice and long. Find your neutral pelvis and spine position.

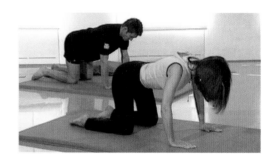

Take a deep breath in and zip up the pelvis, then as you breathe out, slide one leg back keeping the foot in contact with the floor. Breathe in and bring the leg back in again. Repeat with the other leg.

Step 1

Step 2

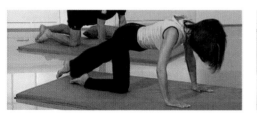

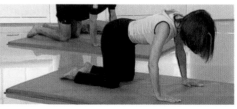

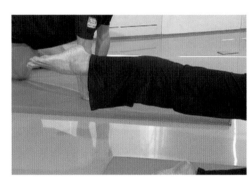

Step 1

To make the above exercise harder, after you have slid the leg back lift it to hip height, hold for a few seconds, then lower the leg and slide it back in. Repeat with the other leg.

Step 2

Step 3

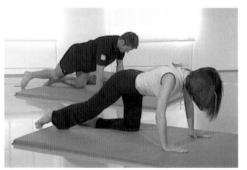

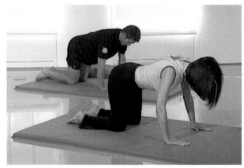

To make the exercise harder still, after you have slid the leg back and lifted it to hip height, bend the knee bringing the foot towards your bottom. Then straighten the leg, lower the leg and bring it back in. The pelvis must stay square and level at all times. You can work up to doing several repetitions on each leg.

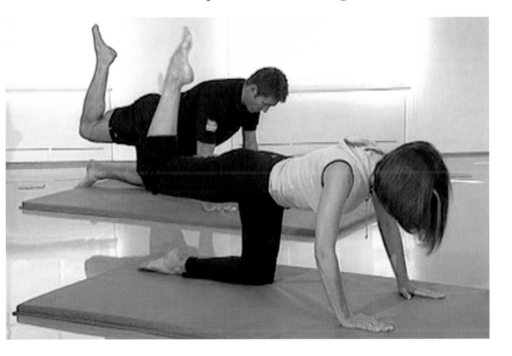

Bring your feet together but leave your knees apart, and slowly lower yourself back down. Rest your forehead onto the mat and stretch out the back taking a few deep breaths. Hold for ten seconds.

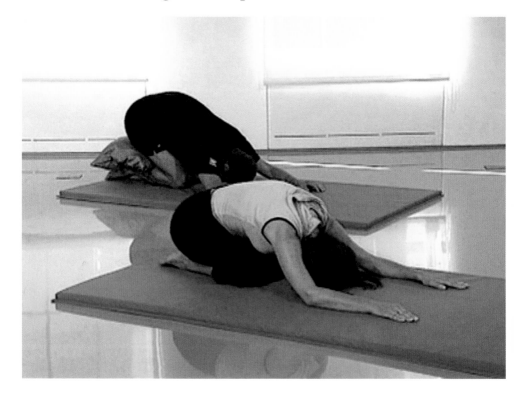

As you breathe out for the last time, bone by bone, bring your pubic bone forward as you roll slowly back up through the spine and then sit up tall.

Step 1

Step 2

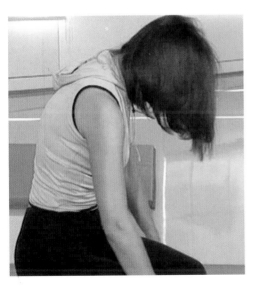 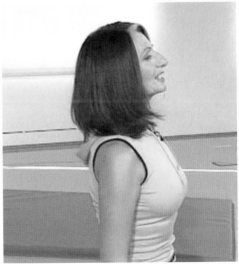

Chapter 11

Spine Curl on Wall with Pillow Squeeze

For this exercise you'll need a non-slip mat placed with its end against a wall. You will also need a plump cushion.

Lie with your knees at a right angle to the wall, your feet together on the wall and all joints lined up in parallel. Place the cushion between your knees and relax back down.

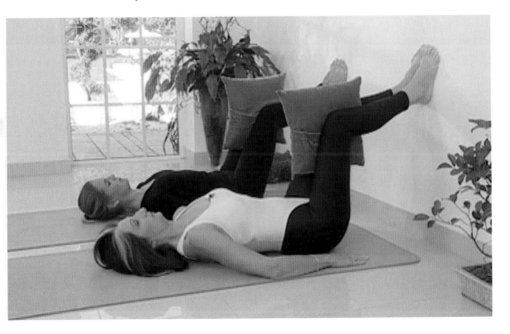

Take a moment to allow your back to lengthen and widen. Take a deep breath in and as you breathe out, zip up the pelvis, squeeze the cushion between the knees and send your tailbone away from you. Bone by bone by bone, curl your spine up away from the mat, squeezing the cushion at all times. Come up to about your shoulder blades and make sure the back of the neck stays long.

Step 1

Step 2

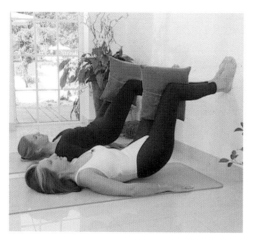
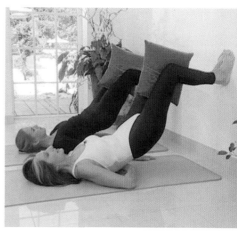

Take a deep breath in at the top and as you breathe out, still zipped, replace the spine, vertebra by vertebra, lengthening through the spine until you come back down to neutral. Repeat twice more.

Step 1

Step 2

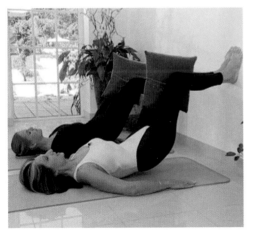

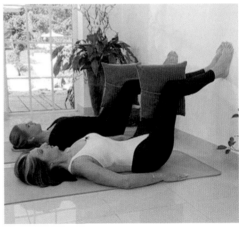

Chapter 12

Gluteal Stretch

This exercise can be done either with or without the aid of a wall.

Lie on your back with one leg up and take the other leg across it, resting just below the knee joint. Keep your pelvis neutral – do not let it twist.

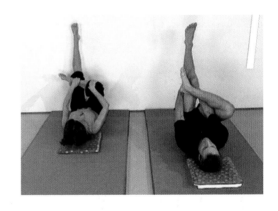

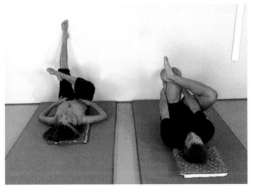

Bend the straight leg back towards you until you feel a stretch on the gluteal on the bent leg side. Hold for several seconds to stretch out. Repeat on the other side.

Chapter 13

Roll Downs

The correct standing position: stand with your feet hip width apart and parallel, making sure that your feet aren't rolling in and out. Knees should be soft, pelvis in its neutral position, long waist and arms relaxed down by your side. Imagine a piece of string attached to the top of your head lengthening you upwards and a little weight in your tailbone just anchoring you at the base of the spine.

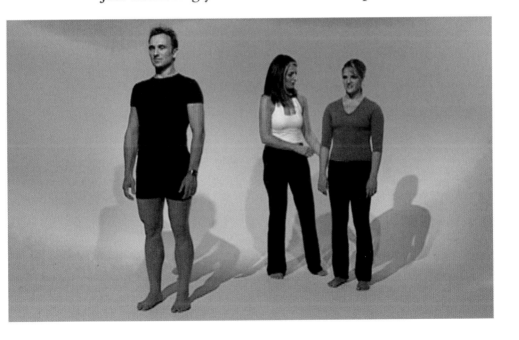

Take a deep breath in, as you breathe out, zip up the pelvis, keep the knees softly bent, tuck your chin in and gently roll forward. Bone by bone by bone, rolling down.

Step 1

Step 2

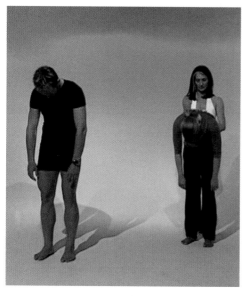 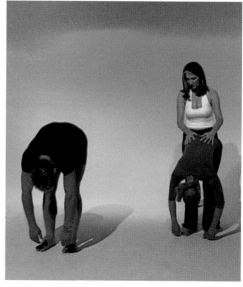

Take a deep breath in at the bottom and as you breathe out bring the pubic bone forward, tuck your tailbone under and restack, bone by bone, to come back up tall. Repeat.

Step 1

Step 2

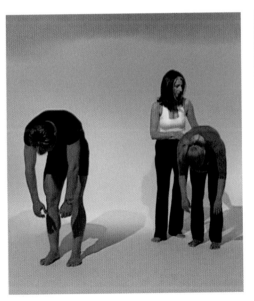

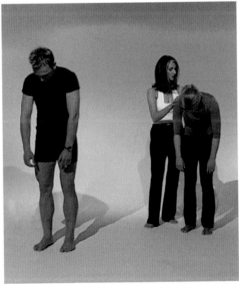

Chapter 14

The Curl Up

Lie on the mat with your feet flat on the floor and make sure that your pelvis is in neutral at all times – don't allow your tailbone to tuck under, keep your pelvis down on the mat and the front of the pelvis stays level with the ceiling. Clasp your hands behind your head with your elbows bent and tuck your chin in gently.

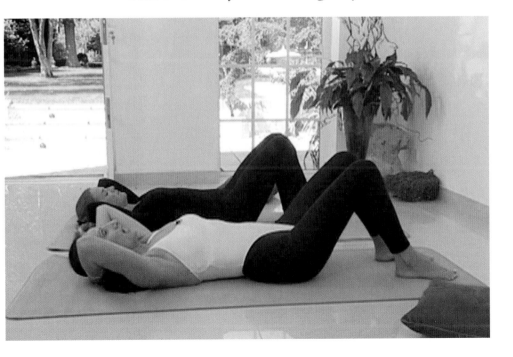

Take a deep breath in to prepare, as you breathe out zip up the pelvis, soften the breastbone and funnel your ribcage down until you've gently curled up.

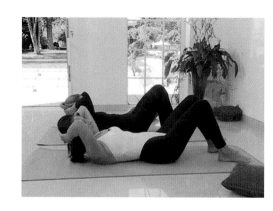

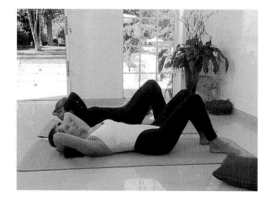

You can either come back down on an in breath, or take an extra in breath while you're up there and come back down on an out breath. Repeat the curl up twice more.

Chapter 15

The Dart

Lying on the mat face down, ensure that you're lying in a straight line. Take your arms down by your sides and you may like to put a flat pillow underneath your forehead to give you a chance to breathe in this position. Your neck should feel really comfortable. Have your toes together and your heels apart.

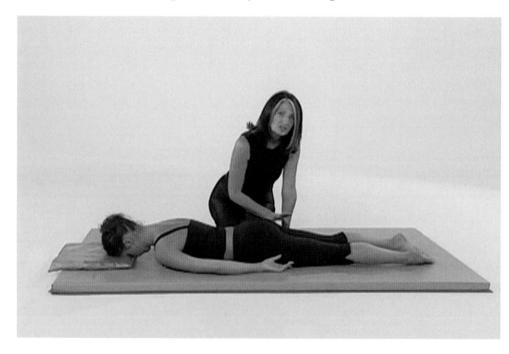

Take a deep breath in to prepare and as you breathe out zip up the pelvis, squeeze the buttocks together, squeeze your inner thighs together, bring your heels together and slide your shoulder blades down your back, turning your palms to face your body. Hold for a few seconds and as you breathe out lengthen and lower back down again. Repeat twice more.

Step 1

Step 2

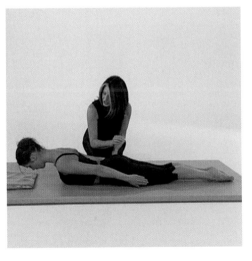

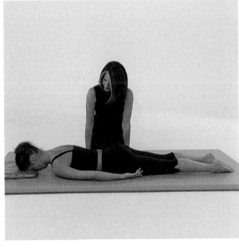

Chapter 16

Double Heel Kicks

To make The Dart a little bit harder, an exercise called Double Heel Kicks can be introduced. This is harder on the back, so stick to The Dart if necessary.

Lie as you were for The Dart, but place your hands on your back.

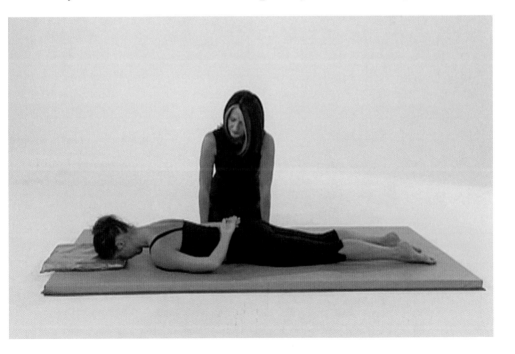

Take a deep breath in to prepare and as you breathe out zip up the pelvis. As you breathe in again kick your feet in towards your bottom three times.

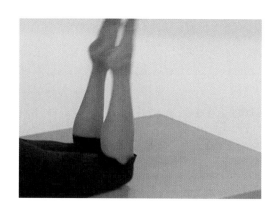

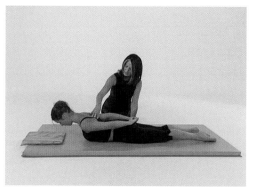

Then as the legs lower, so you come up with the hands and shoulder blades sliding down your body.

As you go back down again, so the feet come up and repeat the above. Do the whole exercise cycle five times.

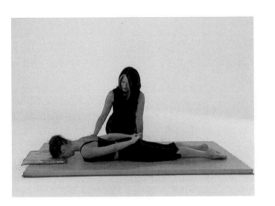

To finish the exercise, come back onto your heels, hold and stretch the lower back for twenty seconds.

On an out breath, slowly curl back up bringing you head up last.

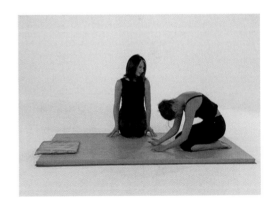

Chapter 17

The Cobra

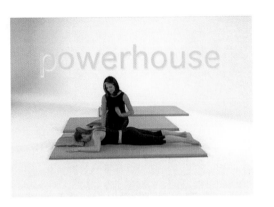

Lie on your front and have your legs turned out and completely relaxed. Have your arms at a right angle, so that the upper part of your arms is level with your shoulders and the lower part of the arm is parallel with each other, with the palms flat.

Take a deep breath and as you breathe out zip up the pelvis, slide your shoulder blades down your back and very slowly bring you upper body back and up.

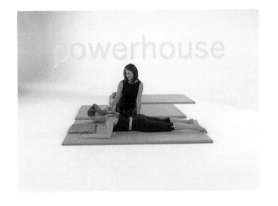

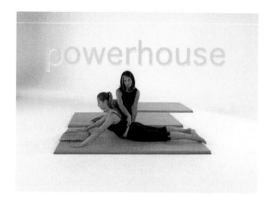

If you like you can, slowly come up a little bit further, but this obviously requires you to have quite a lot of flexibility in your lower back. Anytime you feel your back pinching come back down again. Make sure you continue supporting your back with your lower abdominals.

Breathe in at the top and as you breathe out, very slowly lower back down.

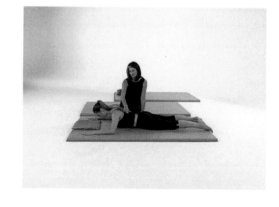

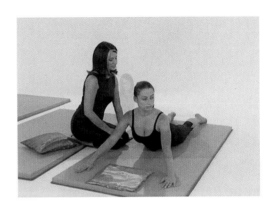

Repeat the above, but this time once at the top, turn your head slowly over one shoulder.

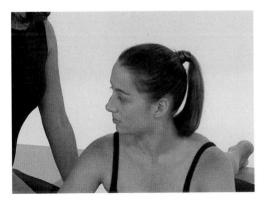

Move back to the centre, turn your head to the other side. Move back to the centre and on the out breath slowly lower back down.

Repeat the exercise with the head turn on each side.

Chapter 18

Mermaid

Sit on the mat on your side and make sure that your knees are in line, and with your feet and hand a little way away from you. Hold on to the front of your shin with the other hand.

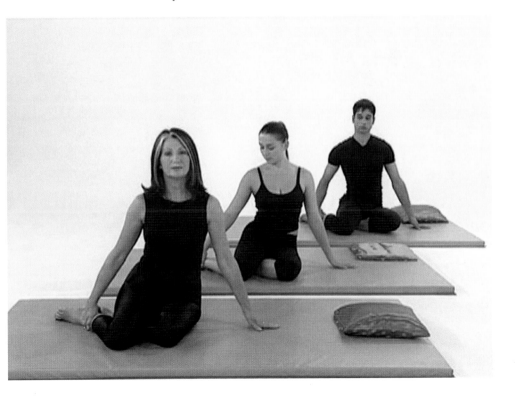

Breathe in to prepare and lengthen through the spine, breathe out and zip up the pelvis. Breathe in and bring the arm up, over and across.

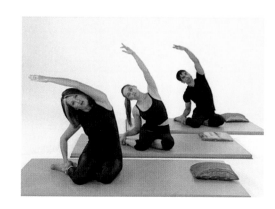

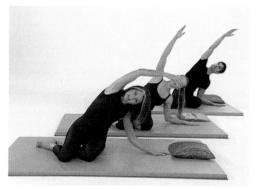

Breathe in as you come up and out as you come down and stretch across the other way.

Repeat the above four more times and then do the exercise on the other side.

Chapter 19

Side Bends

The Mermaid is an excellent preparation exercise for this one; there are two different versions. If you have wrist or shoulder problems you may want to avoid these exercises.

Come onto your side leaning on your elbow with your hand and forearm parallel. Stretch the bottom leg out away from you, slightly in front of your body and take your top leg over with your foot facing forwards. Make sure that you are on your hip and are nice and long through the spine.

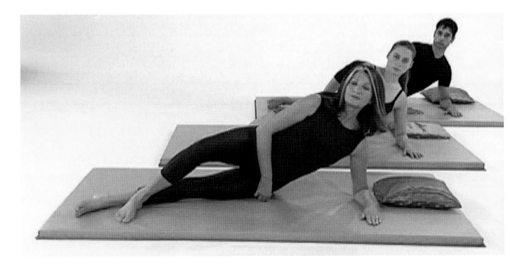

Take a deep breath in to prepare and zip up the pelvis as you breathe out. Stretch up and over making sure that the weight stays on your front foot, which will make it easier. Squeeze your inner thighs together.

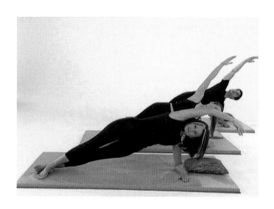

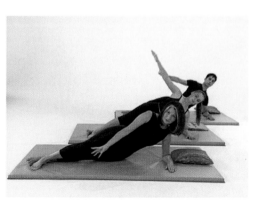

Breathe in as you slowly lower. Repeat the above.

Step 1

The next version you do with a straight arm instead; everything else remains the same.

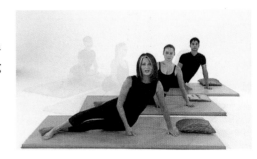

Step 2

Step 3

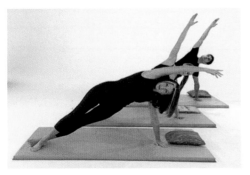

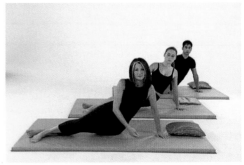

Repeat both versions of Side Bends on the other side.

Chapter 20

Seated Rotation

SEATED ROTATION

Sit cross-legged if it's comfortable, if not then you can try this exercise sitting on a chair. Make sure that you are lengthened through the spine and you are sitting well on your sitting bones. Put your right hand on your left knee and place your left hand behind you.

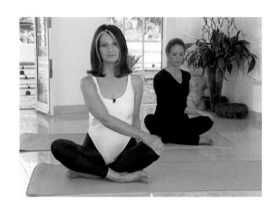

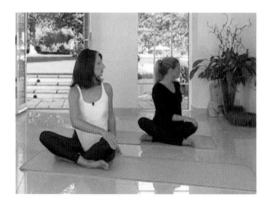

Take a deep breath in to prepare and zip up the pelvis as you breathe out. On the next in breath gently turn to look over your left shoulder. Don't take the head round too far. Take a couple of breaths in this position keeping soft in between your shoulder blades. On the next out breath come back to centre.

Repeat the above but the opposite way round with your left hand on
your knee and your right hand behind you.

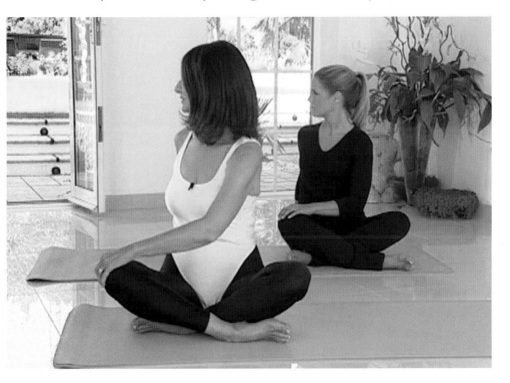

Repeat the exercise one more time on both sides.

Design and artwork by Scott Giarnese

Published by Demand Media Limited

Publishers Jason Fenwick & Jules Gammond

Written by Michelle Brachet